The Ultimate Sirtfood Diet Dinner Cookbook

50 super tasty and super healthy recipes to make your dinner taste delicious!

Anne Patel

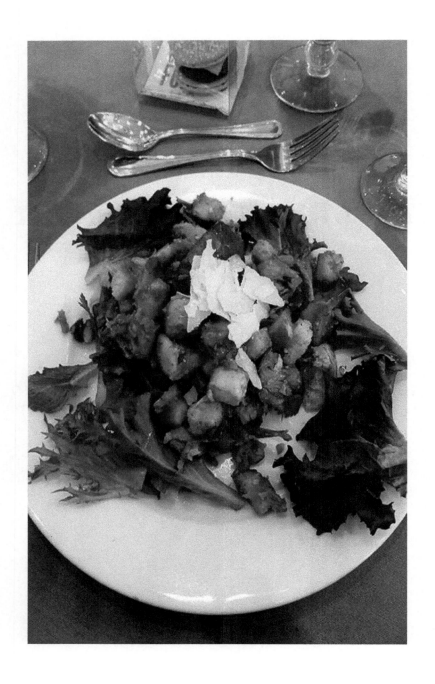

Table of Contents

© Copyright 2021 - All rights reserved. 3

Chapter 1: What is the Sirtfood diet 7

Chapter 2: How do the Sirtfood Diet Works? 16

50 Essential Dinner Recipes 20

1. Beef bourguignon with Mashed Potatoes and Kale 20

2. Turkish fajitas 23

3. Sirt Chicken Korma 26

4. Prawns, Pak Choi and broccoli 28

5. Cocoa spaghetti Bolognese 30

6. Baked salmon with Watercress sauce and Potatoes 32

7. Coq au vin with potatoes and green beans 34

8. Salmon buckwheat Pasta 37

9. Cauliflower Kale curry 39

10. Kidney bean burritos 41

11. Spiced Cauliflower Couscous with Chicken 44

12. Chicken Noodles 46

13. Chicken Butternut Squash Pasta 47

14. Chicken Marsala 50

15. Turkey Apple Burgers 52

16. Turkey Sandwiches with Apple and Walnut Mayo 54

17. Sautéed Turkey with Tomatoes and Cilantro...................56

18. Prawn & Coconut Curry......................................58

19. Orecchiette with Sausage and Chicory.............................59

20. Lamb and Black Bean Chili..61

21. Tomato, Bacon and Arugula Quiche with Sweet Potato Crust 63

22. Pomegranate Guacamole 65

23. Broccoli and Beef Stir-Fry.. 66

24. Meatballs with Eggplant 68

25. Slow-Cooked Lemon Chicken 70

26. Pork with Pak Choi...72

27. Chicken stir-fry...74

28. Tuna with lemon herb dressing 75

29. Kale, apple & fennel soup...76

30. Lentil soup..77

31. Cauliflower & walnut soup 79

32. Celery & blue cheese soup.. 80

33. Spicy squash soup 81

34. French onion soup.. 82

35. Cream of broccoli & kale soup.. 83

36. Sesame miso chicken 84

37. Sirt Salmon Salad..86

38. Red Onion Dhal 87

39. Tofu & Shiitake mushroom soup........................89

40. Chicken Soup... 91

41. Chicken curry with potatoes and kale................93

42. Paleo Chocolate Wraps with Fruits 96

43. Sirt Energy Balls 98

44. Kale and Tofu Curry 99

45. Bean Stew...101

46. Sirt Salmon Salad 103

47. Roasted vegetable salad................................... 105

48. Warm leek and sweet potato salad................... 107

49. Chickpeas, Onion, Tomato & Parsley Salad in a Jar 109

50. Kale & Feta Salad with Cranberry Dressing....................110

Chapter 1: What is the Sirtfood diet

The Sirtfood Diet was created by Masters in Nutritional Medicine, Aiden Goggins and Glen Matten.

Their goal initially was to find a healthier way for people to eat, but people started losing weight quickly when they tested their program. With all the people in the world following diets hoping to lose pounds, they thought it would be selfish not to disclose their innovative health plan.

The plan they developed focuses on combining certain foods eaten in order to maximize the supply of nutrition to our body. There is an initial phase in which calories are limited to give the body a period to recover and eliminate accumulated waste. A maintenance phase follows this first phase to accustom the metabolism to the new foods you are ingesting. Throughout all stages, you will incorporate potent green juices and well-structured, well-planned meals.

The diet focuses on so-called 'sirtfoods,' plant-based foods that are known to stimulate a gene called sirtuin in the human body. Sirtuins belong to an entire protein family, called SIRT1 to SIRT7, and each has specific health-related connections. These proteins help separate and safeguard our cells from inflammation and other damage resulting from everyday activities, helping to reduce our risk of developing major diseases, particularly those related to aging.

Studies have shown that people live longer and healthier lives when they eat diets rich in these foods that activate sirtuin, free from diabetes, heart disease, and even dementia. So this diet was designed to restore a healthy body situation, and one of the byproducts of a healthy body is also the loss of excess weight.

The diet Sirtfood is neither a miracle cure nor a week-long program designed to quickly lose weight before beach holidays. If you are only interested in losing a few pounds and then returning to your old habits, there are certainly plans and diets that are more suited to your needs.

The Sirtfood diet is a project born to help you for the rest of your life, using delicious foods, but that will also improve your health. If you switch from a standard American diet (SAD) to a sirtfood diet, you will lose all the weight your body does not need.

A healthy body does not store extra energy. It asks for what it needs and uses it effectively.

The diet isn't designed to encourage you to starve or deprive yourself. The fact is, foods that are deficient in nutrients are designer made to deprive you and, though the calories are there in plenty, your cells are still starved for the nutrition to help you thrive. The Sirtfood Diet is the opposite of deprivation and starvation. It is nourishment and balance.

Most people following the SAD may use 20 ingredients in a month, let alone enjoy the sheer volume of choice ingredients from the 120 options you will learn about here.

In recent decades, an alarming number of people have come to the conclusion that healthy food is boring, and plants or, more specifically, vegetables are terrible tasting. This is because the foods we've become dependent on – packed with sugar, salt, and unhealthy fats – have chemically altered our connection to food. Our brains are essentially lying to us, and our taste buds have been compromised.

This is one of the reasons the week-long reset is so important. After this first week, you will be able to taste food differently. The more you expose yourself to the recommended plant-based foods, the more pleasure you get out of them.

Sirtuins are critical for our health, regulating many essential biological functions, including our metabolism, which, I'm sure you know, is very closely connected to our weight. It's also a key figure in determining our body composition, such as how much muscle we build and how much fat we retain.

Sirtuin genes regulate all this and more. They're also integral in the process of aging and disease.

If we can turn these genes on, we'll be able to protect our cells and enjoy better health for longer life. Eating sirtfoods is the most effective way to accomplish this goal.

Sirtfoods are all plant-based, and they have many more benefits, in addition to being sirtuin activators.

Our bodies require energy to operate, and the majority of this fuel comes from three primary macronutrients: carbohydrates, fats, and proteins. These macros largely control our metabolic system and regulate how the calories we consume get processed by our bodies. This is why most diets focus exclusively on micronutrition and require you to calculate calories.

Our bodies need more than just energy to survive than thriving, however, which is why micronutrients are so important. They don't impact our weight as obviously as macros, but they are our health foundations.

Micronutrients, such as vitamins, minerals, fiber, antioxidants, and phytonutrients, are supposed to be consumed along with our calories. Unfortunately, in the Standard American Diet (SAD), they're in very limited supply.

When your diet is primarily made up of large quantities of red meat and processed meats, pre-packaged foods, vegetable oils, refined grains and a lot of sugar, you will have an almost total lack of micronutrition.

Plant foods offer the most micronutrients per calorie consumed. Every edible plant has a unique nutritional profile, protecting you from an innumerable variety of illnesses.

Sirtfoods, and other plant-based sources of nutrition, give your body what it needs to stay young and disease-free, and, as a bonus, this will help you remain at an ideal weight.

The original Sirtfood Diet encourages you to commit to a one week reset phase and then a 2-week maintenance phase where you rely heavily on the Sirtfood green juice for a significant dose of nutrition along with meals rich in sirtfoods. Once the phases are complete, to retain your health for the rest of your life, you will need to continue incorporating these sirtfoods into your daily meals.

The Sirtfood Diet is not a miracle cure, but if you stick to these recipes, you'll not just impress your taste buds, but you'll also enhance nearly every aspect of your health. To get safe, you don't have to count calories or starve yourself, the youthful body you've always wanted.

Sirtfood Diet Phases

Every newbie needs to understand that the sirtfood diet does not start with a single list of ingredients in your hands. Its implementation and adaptation are more than mere selective grocery shopping. Every diet can only work effectively when we allow our body to embrace the sudden shift and change in food intake. Similarly, the sirtfood diet also comes with two phases of adaptation. If a dieter successfully goes through these phases, he can continue with the sirtfood diet easily. There are mainly two phases of this diet, which are then succeeded by a third phase in which you can decide how you want to continue the diet.

Phase One

The first seven days of this diet plan are characterized as Phase One. In this phase, a dieter must focus on calorie restriction and the intake of green juices. These seven days are crucial to initiate your weight loss and usually help to lose up to seven pounds if the diet is followed properly. If you find yourself achieving this target, that means that you are on the right track.

In the first three days of the first phase, a dieter must restrict this caloric intake to 1,000 calories only. While doing so, the dieter must also have green juice throughout the day, probably three times a day. Try to drink green juice per meal. The recipes given in the book are perfect for selecting from.

Many meal options can keep your caloric intake in checks, such as buckwheat noodles, seared tofu, some shrimp stir fry, or sirtfood omelet.

Once the first three days of this diet has passed, you can increase your caloric intake to 1,500 calories per day. In these next four days, you can reduce the green juices to two times per side. And pair the juices with more Sirtuin-rich food in every meal.

Phase Two

After the first week of the sirtfood diet, then starts phase two. This phase is more about the maintenance of the diet, as the first week enables the body to embrace the change and start working according to the new diet. This phase enables the body to continue working towards the weight loss objective slowly and steadily. Therefore, the duration of this phase is almost two weeks.

So how is this phase different from phase one? In this phase, there is no restriction on the caloric intake, as long as the food is rich in sirtuins and you are taking it three times a day, it is good to go. Instead of having the green juice two or three times a day, the dieter can have juice one time a day, and that will be enough to achieve steady weight loss. You can have the juice after any meal, in the morning or in the evening.

After the Diet Phase

With the end of phase two comes the time, which is most crucial, and that is the after-diet phase. If your weight loss target has not been reached by the end of step two, then you can restart the phases all over again. Or even when you have achieved the goals but still want to lose more weight, then you can again give it a try.

Instead of following phases one and two over and over again, you can also continue having good quality sirtfood meals in this after-diet phase. Simply continue the eating practices of phase two, have a diet rich in sirtuin and do have green juices whenever possible. The diet is mainly divided into two phases: the first lasts one week, and the other lasts 14 days.

The best 20 sirt foods

All these foods include high quantities of plant compounds called polyphenols, which can be thought to modify the sirtuin enzymes, therefore, excite their super-healthy added benefits.

Top 20 sirtfoods

1. Arugula (Rocket)
2. Buckwheat
3. Capers
4. Celery
5. Chilis
6. Cocoa
7. Coffee
8. Extra Virgin Olive Oil
9. Garlic
10. Green Tea (especially Matcha)
11. Kale
12. Medjool Dates
13. Parsley
14. Red Endive
15. Red Onions
16. Red Wine
17. Soy
18. Strawberries
19. Turmeric
20. Walnuts

What Is So Great About Sirtuins?

There are seven types of Sirtuins named from **SIRT1** to **SIRT7**. Although our understanding of the exact functions of all the Sirtuins is minimal, studies show that activating them can have the following benefits:

Switching on fat burning and protection from weight gain: Sirtuins do this by increasing the mitochondrion's functionality (which is involved in the production of energy) and sparking a change in your metabolism to break down more fat cells.

Improving Memory by protecting neurons from damage. Sirtuins also boost learning skills and memory through the enhancement of synaptic plasticity. Synaptic plasticity refers to synapses' capacity to weaken or strengthen with time due to decreased or increased activity. This is important because memories are represented by different interconnected networks of synapses in the brain, and synaptic plasticity is an important neurochemical foundation of memory and learning.

Slowing down the Ageing Process: Sirtuins act as cell guarding enzymes. Thus, they protect the cells and slow down their aging process.

Repairing cells: The Sirtuins repair cells damaged by re-activating cell functionality.

Protection against diabetes: this happens through prevention against insulin resistance. Sirtuins do this by controlling blood sugar levels because this diet calls for moderate consumption of carbohydrates. These foods cause increases in blood sugar levels; hence the need to release insulin, and as the blood sugar levels increase greatly, there is a need to produce more insulin.

Over time, cells become resistant to insulin, hence producing more insulin and leading to insulin resistance.

Fighting Cancers: The chemicals working as sirtuin activators affect the function of sirtuin in different cells, i.e. by switching it on when in normal cells and shutting it down in cancerous cells. This encourages the death of cancerous cells.

Fighting inflammation: Sirtuins have a powerful antioxidant effect that has the power to reduce oxidative stress. This has positive effects on heart health and cardiovascular protection.

Chapter 2: How do the Sirtfood Diet Works?

The basis of the sirtuin diet can be explained in simple terms or in complex ways. However, it's important to understand how and why it works so that you can appreciate the value of what you are doing. It is important to also know why these sirtuin rich foods help to help you maintain fidelity to your diet plan. Otherwise, you may throw something in your meal with less nutrition that would defeat the purpose of planning for one rich in sirtuins. Most importantly, this is not a dietary fad, and as you will see, there is much wisdom contained in how humans have used natural foods, even for medicinal purposes, over thousands of years.

To understand how the Sirtfood diet works and why these particular foods are necessary, we're going to look at their role in the human body.

Sirtuin activity was first researched in yeast, where a mutation caused an extension in the yeast's lifespan. Sirtuins were also shown to slow aging in laboratory mice, fruit flies, and nematodes. As research on Sirtuins proved to transfer to mammals, they were examined for their use in diet and slowing the aging process. The sirtuins in humans are different in typing, but they essentially work in the same ways and reasons.

The Sirtuin family is made up of seven "members." It is believed that sirtuins play a big role in regulating certain functions of cells, including proliferation, reproduction and growth of cells), apoptosis death of cells). They promote survival and resist stress to increase longevity.

They are also seen to block neurodegeneration loss or function of the nerve cells in the brain). They conduct their housekeeping functions by cleaning out toxic proteins and supporting the brain's ability to change and adapt to different conditions or to recuperate i.e., brain plasticity). They also help minimize chronic inflammation as part of this and decrease anything called oxidative stress. Oxidative stress is when there are so many free radicals present in the body that are cell-damaging, and by fighting them with antioxidants, the body can not keep up. These factors are related to age-related illness and weight as well, which again brings us back to a discussion of how they actually work.

You will see labels in Sirtuins that start with "SIR," which represents "Silence Information Regulator" genes. They do exactly that, silence or regulate, as part of their functions. Humans work with the seven sirtuins: SIRT1, SIRT2, SIRT3, SIRT4, SIRT 5, SIRT6 and SIRT7. Each of these types is responsible for different areas of protecting cells. They work by either stimulating or turning on certain gene expressions or by reducing and turning off other gene expressions. This essentially means that they can influence genes to do more or less of something, most of which they are already programmed to do.

Through enzyme reactions, each of the SIRT types affects different areas of cells responsible for the metabolic processes that help maintain life. This is also related to what organs and functions they will affect.

For example, the SIRT6 causes and expression of genes in humans that affect skeletal muscle, fat tissue, brain, and heart. SIRT 3 would cause an expression of genes that affect the kidneys, liver, brain and heart.

If we tie these concepts together, you can see that the Sirtuin proteins can change the expression of genes, and in the case of the Sirtfood diet, we care about how sirtuins can turn off those genes that are responsible for speeding up aging and for weight management.

The other aspect to this conversation of sirtuins is the function and the power of calorie restriction on the human body. Calorie restriction is simply eating fewer calories. This, coupled with exercise and reducing stress, is usually a combination for weight loss. Calorie restriction has also proven across much research in animals and humans to increase one's lifespan.

We can look further at the role of sirtuins with calorie restriction and using the SIRT3 protein, which has a role in metabolism and aging. Amongst all of the effects of the protein on gene expression, such as preventing cells from dying, reducing tumors from growing, etc.), we want to understand the effects of SIRT3 on weight for this book's purpose.

As we stated earlier, the SIRT3 has high expression in those metabolically active tissues, and its ability to express itself increases with caloric restriction, fasting, and exercise. On the contrary, it will express itself less when the body has high fat, high calorie-riddled diet.

The last few highlights of sirtuins are their role in regulating telomeres and reducing inflammation, which also helps with staving off disease and aging. Telomeres are sequences of proteins at the ends of chromosomes. When cells divide, these get shorter. As we age, they get shorter, and other stressors to the body also will contribute to this. Maintaining these longer telomeres is the key to slower aging. In addition, proper diet, along with exercise and other variables, can lengthen telomeres. SIRT6 is one of the sirtuins that, if activated, can help with DNA damage, inflammation and oxidative stress. SIRT1 also helps with inflammatory response cycles that are related to many age-related diseases.

Calories restriction can extend life to some degree. Since this and fasting are a stressor, these factors will stimulate the SIRT3 proteins to kick in and protect the body from the stressors and excess free radicals. Again, the telomere length is affected as well.

Having laid this all out before you, you should appreciate how and why these miraculous compounds work in your favor, keep you youthful, healthy, and lean If they are working hard for you, don't you feel that you should do something too?

50 Essential Dinner Recipes

1. Beef bourguignon with Mashed Potatoes and Kale

Preparation time: 15 minutes.
Cooking time: 2–3 hours.
Serving: 4

Ingredients:

800 grams diced beef

1 tablespoon extra-virgin olive oil

150 grams red onion, roughly chopped

200 grams celery, roughly chopped

100 grams carrots, roughly chopped

2–3 cloves of garlic, chopped

375 milliliters of red wine

2 tablespoon tomato puree

750 milliliters beef broth

2 bay leaves

1 sprig of fresh thyme or 1 tablespoon of dried thyme

75 grams diced pancetta or smoked lard

250 grams mushrooms

2 tablespoon chopped parsley

200 grams kale

1 tablespoon cornflour or arrowroot (optional)

For the porridge:

500 grams Edward potatoes

1 tablespoon milk and 1 tablespoon olive oil

Directions:

1. Pat the beef dry with kitchen paper. Heat a heavy saucepan over medium-high heat. Add the olive oil, then the beef and saute the meat until completely browned. Depending on the size of your pan, it's best to do this in 3– 4 small loads.

2. When all of the meat is brown, remove it from the pan with a slotted spoon and set aside. Add the onion, celery, carrot and garlic to the same pan and fry for 3 to 4 minutes over medium heat until tender. Add the wine, tomato paste and broth and bring to a boil. Add the browned beef, bay leaves and thyme and reduce the heat to a simmer. Cover the pan with a lid and cook for 2 hours to ensure that nothing sticks to the rim, stirring from time to time. While the beef is cooking, peel your potatoes and cut them into quarters (or smaller pieces if they're quite large).

3. Put in a pan with cold water and bring to a boil. Reduce the heat to a simmer and cook for 20–25 minutes, covered with a lid. When soft, drain and mash with olive oil and milk. Keep warm. While the potatoes are boiling, heat a pan over high heat. Then add the diced pancetta when it's hot but not smoking.

4. The fat content of the bacon means you don't need oil to cook it. Once some of the fat is released and it begins to brown, add the mushrooms and cook over medium heat until both are nicely browned. Depending on the size of your pan, you may need to do this in multiple loads. Set aside after cooking. Cook or steam the kale for 5–10 minutes until soft. Once the beef is tender enough and the sauce has thickened to your liking, add the pancetta,

mushrooms, and parsley. If your sauce is always kind of runny, you can mix the cornflour or arrowroot with a little water and then stir the paste into the sauce until you have the consistency you want. Cook for 2-3 minutes and serve with porridge and kale.

Nutrition
Carbohydrates: 34g
Fat: 25g
Protein: 31g
Kcal: 510cal

2. Turkish fajitas

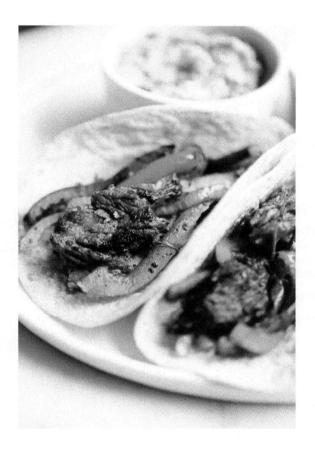

Preparation time: 15 minutes.

Cooking time: approx. 1 hour.

Serving: 4

Ingredients:

For the filling:

500 grams turkey breast into strips

1 tablespoon of extra virgin olive oil 1–2 chilies, depending on taste, chopped

150 grams red onion, thinly sliced

150 grams red pepper, cut into thin strips 2–3 cloves of garlic, chopped

1 tablespoon paprika

1 tablespoon ground cumin

1 teaspoon chili powder

1 tablespoon chopped coriander

For the guacamole:

2 ripe avocados, peeled (reserve one of the stones)

Juice of 1 lime

Pinch of chili powder

Pinch of black pepper

For the salsa:

1×400 grams can of chopped tomatoes 20 grams red onion, diced

20 grams red pepper, deseeded and diced Juice of ½–1 lime, depending on the size 1 teaspoon chopped coriander

1 teaspoon capers

For the salad:

100 grams rocket

3 tomatoes, cut

100 grams cucumber, thinly sliced

1 tablespoon extra-virgin olive oil juice of ½ lemon

For serving:

100 grams cheddar cheese

8 grated whole grain tortilla wraps

Directions:

1. Mix together the filling ingredients and set them aside while the other parts are prepared.

2. In a small food processor, bring all the guacamole ingredients in and flash until a smooth paste is formed. Alternatively, you can mash them all together with the back of a fork or spoon.

3. Place the reserved avocado stone in the guacamole—it will keep it from turning brown. Mix all the ingredients for the salsa.

4. Put all the salad ingredients in a large tub. Put your largest pan on high heat until it starts to smoke.

5. Put the turkey filling in the hot pan - you may need to cook it in 2 to 3 loads as overcrowding the pan will create too much moisture and it will start boiling instead of frying.

6. Keep the pan over high heat and keep moving the mixture, so the turkey colors nicely but doesn't burn.

7. In a low oven, keep the cooked meat warm. To serve, reheat the tortillas according to the directions in the package, then sprinkle some guacamole over each package.

8. Top with some cheese and some salsa, then stack the turkey mixture in the middle and roll it up like a large cigar. Serve with the salad.

Nutrition
Carbohydrates: 44g
Fat: 21g

Protein: 30g

Kcal: 450cal

3. Sirt Chicken Korma

Preparation time: 10 minutes
Cooking time: 50 minutes
Serving: 4

Ingredients:
350 ml chicken stock
30 g Medjool date, chopped
2 cinnamon sticks
4–5 cardamom pods, slightly split 250 ml coconut milk
8 boneless, skinless chicken thighs
1 tablespoon ground turmeric
200 g buckwheat
150 ml of Greek yogurt
50 g of ground walnuts
2 tablespoon chopped coriander

For the curry paste
1 large red onion, quartered
3 cloves of garlic
2 cm piece of fresh ginger
1 tbsp mild curry powder
1 teaspoon ground cumin
1 tbsp ground turmeric
1 tbsp coconut oil

Directions

1. In a food processor, place the ingredients for the curry paste and flash for about a minute until you have a nice paste.

2. Alternatively, you can use a pestle and mortar to grind it. Fry the paste in a heavy pan over medium heat for 1-2 minutes then add the broth, date, cinnamon, cardamom pods, and coconut milk.

3. Bring to a boil then add the chicken legs. Reduce the heat, cover the pan with a lid, and simmer for 45 minutes.

4. Meanwhile, bring it to a boil with a pan of water and whisk in the turmeric.

5. Add the buckwheat and cook according to the directions on the package. As soon as the chicken is tender, stir in the yogurt and cook the walnuts over low heat for a few more minutes.

6. Add the coriander and serve with the buckwheat

Nutrition
Carbohydrates: 21
Fat: 16
Protein: 32
Kcal: 330

4. Prawns, Pak Choi and broccoli

Preparation time: 15 minutes
Cooking time: 20 minutes
Serving: 5

Ingredients:
1 tbsp ground turmeric
400 g raw shrimp, peeled and deveined
1 tbsp coconut oil
280 g buckwheat noodles
1 teaspoon virgin olive oil
For the china pan
1 tbsp coconut oil
Cut 250 g broccoli into bite-sized pieces 250 g pak choi, roughly chopped 1 red onion, thinly sliced
2 cm piece of fresh ginger, chopped 1–2 chili peppers, chopped
3 cloves of garlic, chopped
150 ml vegetable broth
1 bunch of basil, removed leaves and chopped stems
1 tbsp Thai fish sauce or tamari

Directions
Mix the turmeric with the prawns. Place the coconut oil in a wok or pan and cook the shrimp over medium-high heat for a time of 3 to 4 minutes or until it is opaque.

After cooking, remove from pan and set aside. Wipe the pan for the pan and put it on high heat until it starts to smoke.

Add the coconut oil then add the vegetables, ginger, chili peppers, and garlic.

Keep moving the vegetables in the pan so they don't burn. Cook for 3–5 minutes - lower the heat a little if the vegetables look charred - until they are fried but crispy.

Add the broth, whole basil and fish sauce.

Bring to the boil, then add the shrimp and let heat. In the meantime, cook the pasta according to the instructions on the package.

Freshen up in cold water and mix with the olive oil to prevent them from sticking together. Serve the pan with the hot noodles.

Nutrition
Carbohydrates: 13
Fat: 15
Protein: 26
Kcal: 270

5. Cocoa spaghetti Bolognese

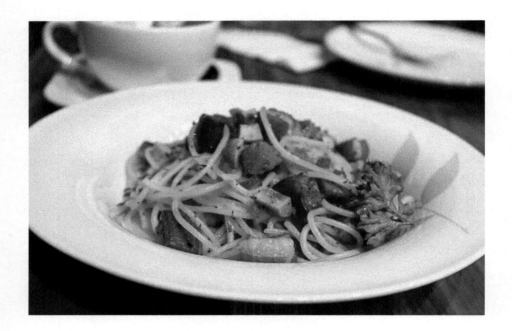

Preparation time: 15 minutes
Cooking time: approx. 1 hour
Serving: 4

Ingredients:
1 tbsp virgin olive oil
1 red onion, finely diced
100 g celery, finely diced
100 g carrots, finely diced
3 cloves of garlic, chopped
400 g of lean ground beef
1 tbsp Herbs de Provence
1–2 bay leaves

150 ml red wine

300 ml beef broth

1 tbsp cocoa powder

1 tbsp tomato paste

2 × 400 g cans of chopped tomatoes

280 g whole wheat spaghetti

1 teaspoon ground black pepper

1 bunch of fresh basil

20 g parmesan cheese

Directions

Heat the oil in a pan and then cook the onion, celery, carrot and garlic over medium heat for 1-2 minutes until they are a little softer.

Add the ground beef and dried herbs and cook over medium-high heat until the ground beef is brown.
Add the wine, stock, cocoa powder, tomato paste and canned tomatoes, bring to a boil and simmer for 45 to 60 minutes with the lid closed.

When you're almost done, cook the pasta as directed on the package.

Finally stir the pepper and basil leaves into the sauce. Serve with the pasta and rub some parmesan on top.

Nutrition

Carbohydrates: 43

Fat: 21

Protein: 11

Kcal: 450

6. Baked salmon with Watercress sauce and Potatoes

Preparation time: 10 minutes
Cooking time: 35 minutes
Serving: 4

Ingredients:
400 g of new potatoes
4 × 125 g skinless salmon fillets
1 teaspoon extra virgin olive oil
1 piece of broccoli, cut into florets
1 bunch of asparagus spears

For the watercress sauce
30 g of watercress
5 g parsley
1 tbsp capers
2 tbsp virgin olive oil
Extra juice of 1 lemon

Directions
Heat the oven to 200 ° C / gas. 6. Place the potatoes with cold water in a tub.

Bring to a boil and simmer for 15-20 minutes or until tender.

Brush the olive oil with the salmon fillets, put them on a baking sheet and bake for 10 minutes in the oven.

When you like your salmon to be lightly cooked, reduce the cooking time by 2 to 3 minutes.

In the meantime, cook or steam the broccoli and asparagus until tender.

Put the ingredients for the sauce in a food processor or blender and stir until smooth. Serve the salmon with the sauce and the vegetables.

Nutrition
Carbohydrates: 9
Fat: 15
Protein: 31
Kcal: 250

7. Coq au vin with potatoes and green beans

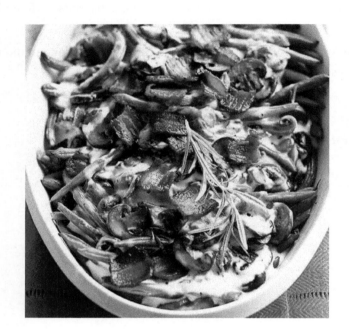

Preparation time: 10 minutes
Cooking time: 35 minutes
Serving: 4

Ingredients:

4 skinless chicken legs

4 skinless chicken legs

1-2 tbsp buckwheat flour

1 tbsp extra virgin olive oil

150 g red onion

150 g carrot

200 g celery

3 cloves of garlic, chopped

400 ml red wine

400 ml of chicken broth

1 sprig of fresh thyme

2–3 bay leaves

100 g pancetta or smoked bacon, diced

250 g mushrooms

400 g of new potatoes

2 tbsp chopped parsley

250 g green beans

Directions

Roll the chicken pieces in the flour. Heat a heavy saucepan over medium-high heat. Then add the olive oil and the chicken and cook until all is nicely browned.

Remove and set aside from the pan. Add the onion, carrot, celery and garlic to the same pan and cook gently for 2-3 minutes until softened.

When the pan is dry, you can add some water here. Add the wine and chicken stock and bring to a boil. Add the thyme, bay leaves, and chicken. Cover and simmer gently for 45 minutes with a lid.

Check the amount of fluid from time to time and add a little more. Heat a pan over high heat. Then add the diced pancetta when it's hot but not smoking.

Once some of the fat is released and it begins to brown, add the mushrooms and cook over medium heat until both it and the pancetta are nicely browned.

Depending on the size of your pan, you may need to do this in multiple loads. Set aside after cooking.

Using cold water to place the potatoes in a tub. Bring to a boil and simmer for 15-20 minutes or until tender. When you're done, drain it and return to the pan to keep it warm.

Add the pancetta, mushrooms and parsley to the Coq au Vin and cook for another 15 minutes.

To cook the green beans, steam them or cook them for 4 to 6 minutes, depending on how crispy you like them.

With the potatoes and beans, serve the Coq au Vin.

Nutrition
Carbohydrates: 13
Fat: 15
Protein: 26
Kcal: 270

8. Salmon buckwheat Pasta

Preparation time: 10 minutes
Cooking time: 25 minutes
Serving: 4

Ingredients:
300 g skinless salmon fillet
1 teaspoon extra virgin olive oil
250 g buckwheat noodles
100 g kale, chopped
1 large zucchini, quarter lengthways
Cut 1 red onion into slices
Cut 4 cloves of garlic into slices
1 tbsp Herbs of Provence
1 tbsp extra virgin olive oil

For the sauce
650 ml milk or dairy-free alternative
65 g unsalted butter
65 g buckwheat or flour
150 g cheddar cheese, grated
2 tbsp chopped parsley
2 tbsp capers

Directions
Heat the oven to 200 ° C / gas. 6. Rub the salmon with olive oil and put it on a piece of foil.

Fold over the edges and seal them to get a package. Bake in the oven for 15 minutes.

Cook the pasta on the box according to the instructions. Drain, then pour some warm water out of the kettle to prevent it from sticking and put aside.

To make the sauce, bring the milk to a boil in a small saucepan, being careful not to overflow it.

Then melt the butter and add it to a separate pan. Mix them together until you have a mixture.

Cook gently over low heat for 30 seconds to 1 minute. Gradually add the hot milk, stirring continuously, until you have a nice thick sauce.

Add 100 g cheese, parsley and capers and remove from heat.

In the meantime, cook or steam the kale until tender.

Cook the zucchini in a pan over medium heat, red onion, garlic and herbs in the olive oil for 2-3 minutes until tender. Mix with the cooked kale.

Heat a grill on the highest setting. Peel the cooked salmon and mix with the pasta, cooked vegetables and sauce, place in an ovenproof bowl and sprinkle over the remaining cheese.

Place under the hot grill for 5 minutes until the cheese turns brown.

Nutrition
Carbohydrates: 13
Fat: 15
Protein: 26
Kcal: 270

9. Cauliflower Kale curry

Preparation time: 10 minutes
Cooking time: 30 minutes
Serving: 4

Ingredients:
200 g buckwheat
2 tbsp ground turmeric
1 red onion, chopped
3 cloves of garlic, minced
2.5 cm piece of fresh ginger, chopped
1–2 chili peppers, chopped
1 tbsp coconut oil
1 tbsp mild curry powder
1 tbsp ground cumin
2 × 400 g cans of chopped tomatoes
300 ml vegetable broth
200 g kale, roughly chopped
300 g cauliflower, chopped
1 × 400 g can of butter beans, drained
2 tomatoes, cut into wedges
2 tbsp chopped coriander

Directions
Cook the buckwheat and add 1 tablespoon of turmeric to the water, as per the directions on the package.

In the meantime, cook the onion, garlic, ginger and chili peppers in the coconut oil over medium heat for 2-3 minutes.

Add the seasonings, including the remaining tablespoon of turmeric and continue cooking over low to medium heat for 1–2 minutes.

Add the canned tomatoes and the broth and bring to a boil then simmer for 10 minutes.

Add the kale, cauliflower and butter beans and cook for 10 minutes.

Add the tomato wedges and coriander and cook for another minute.

Then serve them with the buckwheat.

Nutrition

Carbohydrates: 43

Fat: 21

Protein: 11

Kcal: 450

10. Kidney bean burritos

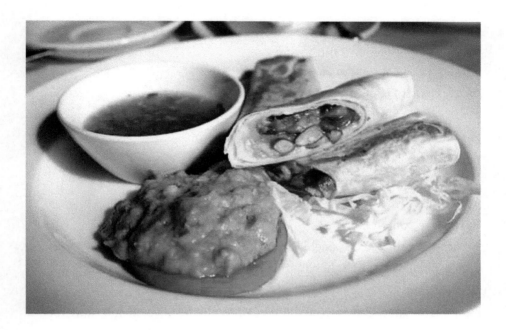

Preparation time: 15 minutes
Cooking time: 45 minutes
Serving: 4

Ingredients:

1 tbsp extra virgin olive oil

1 red onion, diced

3 cloves of garlic, chopped

1 tablespoon chili, chopped

1 tbsp paprika

1 tbsp ground cumin

1 teaspoon chili powder

1 tbsp chopped coriander

2 tomatoes, chopped

3 × 400 g cans of kidney beans, drained

500 ml vegetable broth

150 g cheddar or vegan cheese

8 whole grain tortilla wraps

1 × 500 g glass of tomato passata

1 × 200 g jar of jalepeño peppers (optional)

For the salad:

125 g rocket

1 paprika,

3 tomatoes sliced,

½ small red onion sliced

1 avocado cut into slices, peeled and sliced

1 tablespoon of extra virgin olive oil juice ½ lemon

Directions

Heat a large saucepan over medium heat. Apply the olive oil and sauté for 1-2 minutes with the onion, garlic and chili, until slightly softer.

Add the coriander and spices and cook for another 1–2 minutes. Add the tomatoes, kidney beans and broth. Bring to a boil and cook over medium-high heat for 20 minutes.

You want most of the liquid to evaporate. So keep an eye out for them and stir sometimes.

Take off the stove and let cool down a bit. Take about a third of the kidney beans out of the pan and set aside. In a food processor or blender, soften the remaining mixture, then return to the pan, add the whole beans and stir in.

The mixture should be a little stiff. Allowing it to cool fully would make wrapping the burritos easier. Heat the oven to 200 ° C / gas. 6th

Spread the cheese on top of the wraps, holding back a little to spread over the top at the end. Divide the filling and roll each into a sausage tin between the wraps.

Spread a thin layer of passata on the bottom of an ovenproof bowl large enough to hold all of the burritos in a single layer.

Put them in this way and drizzle the rest of the passata over them.

Sprinkle with the remaining cheese and the jalepeños, if used.

Cover the bowl with foil and bake in the oven for 20-25 minutes. Remove the foil and bake for another 5 minutes to brown the cheese.

Throw all the salad ingredients together and serve with the hot burritos.

Nutrition
Carbohydrates: 43
Fat: 21
Protein: 11
Kcal: 450

11. Spiced Cauliflower Couscous with Chicken

Preparation time: 15 minutes
Cooking time: 20 minutes
Servings: 2

Ingredients:
2 cups roughly chopped cauliflower florets
A handful fresh flat-leaf parsley
2 cloves garlic, finely chopped
½ cup finely chopped red onions
2 teaspoons finely chopped ginger
1/3 cup sun-dried tomatoes
2 tablespoons capers
2 chicken breasts
4 teaspoons turmeric powder
½ cup finely diced carrots
2 bird's eye chilies, finely chopped
4 tablespoons extra-virgin olive oil
Juice of a lemon

Directions:
1. You can chop the cauliflower in a food processor.

2. Place a pan over medium – high flame. Add 2 tablespoons oil. When the oil is warmed, add the ginger, the garlic and the chili and cook until fragrant for a few seconds.

3. Stir in turmeric and cook for 5 – 8 seconds. Stir in the carrots and cauliflower and cook for about 2 minutes. Turn off the heat.
4. Transfer into a bowl. Add tomatoes and parsley and stir. Keep warm.

5. Add remaining oil into the pan and let it heat. Place chicken in the pan and cook for about 6 minutes. Turn over the chicken and cook for 5 to 6 minutes or until the inside is well-cooked.

6. Stir in capers, lemon juice and a sprinkle of water.

7. Add cauliflower and carrot mixture and toss well.

8. Serve.

Nutrition: Calories: 250 Fat: 4.5g Protein: 68g Total Carbohydrates: 13g Dietary Fiber: 5g Sodium: 532mg

12. Chicken Noodles

Preparation time: 10 minutes

Cooking time: 30 minutes

Servings: 8 – 10

Ingredients:

16 ounces buckwheat noodles

2 yellow bell peppers, chopped into ½ inch squares

6 cloves garlic, chopped

2 tablespoons olive oil

6 cups tomato sauce

2 tablespoons fresh basil, chopped or 2 teaspoons dry basil

2 tablespoons fresh parsley, chopped or 2 teaspoons dried parsley

Pepper to taste

2 pounds skinless, boneless chicken breast, cut into strips

1 large red onion, chopped into ½ inch squares, separate the layers

Salt to taste

Directions:

1. On the box, follow the instructions and cook the buckwheat noodles.

2. Place a large skillet over medium flame. Add the oil and wait until the oil is hot. Add chicken strips and spread it all over the pan and cook undisturbed, until the underside is cooked. Flip sides and cook the other side, undisturbed.

3. Add the vegetables and mix well. Cook until the vegetables are tender. Add tomato sauce and cook for 7-8 minutes.

4. Add noodles and toss well.

5. Serve hot.

Nutrition: Calories 372.3 Total Fat 12.4 g Protein 42.6 g Carbs 26.1 g

13. Chicken Butternut Squash Pasta

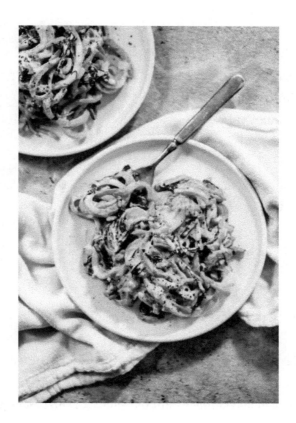

Preparation time: 10 minutes

Cooking time: 30 – 40 minutes

Servings: 2

Ingredients:

½ pound ground chicken

tablespoon balsamic vinegar

½ tablespoon olive oil, divided

½ cups whole wheat pasta

Pepper to taste

fresh basil leaves, thinly sliced

tablespoons chopped walnuts

Salt to taste

½ cups cubed butternut squash, cut into ½" cubes

ounces goat's cheese, crumbled

½ teaspoon garlic, minced

1/8 teaspoon ground nutmeg

Directions:

1 Place butternut squash on a baking sheet. Drizzle 1 tablespoon oil and sprinkle salt and pepper over the squash. Toss well.

2 Bake squash in an oven preheated to 400° F, for about 30 minutes or until tender.

3 Following the package instructions, cook the pasta.

4 Place a skillet over medium heat. Add ½ tablespoon oil and wait for it to heat. Add garlic and cook until light brown, stirring often.
5 Attach the chicken and simmer until the chicken is no longer pink.

6 Stir in walnuts, nutmeg and vinegar.

7 Cook on low heat for 1 – 2 minutes.

8 Serve chicken over pasta.

9 Scatter butternut squash and goat's cheese. Sprinkle basil on top.

Nutrition: Sodium: 198 mg Cholesterol: 0.0 mg Total Carbs: 39.0 g Fiber:

15.0 g Protein: 12.0 g Calories: 247.0

14. Chicken Marsala

Preparation time: 10 minutes
Cooking time: 30 – 40 minutes
Servings: 8

Ingredients:
8 boneless, skinless breasts of chicken (6 ounces each)
20 ounces cremini mushrooms, sliced
2 cloves garlic, peeled, sliced
1 cup marsala wine
6 tablespoons flour
2 large shallots, chopped
Salt to taste
1 cup chicken broth
Freshly ground pepper to taste
4 – 5 tablespoons olive oil
2 tablespoons chopped parsley
Sautéed spinach to serve

Directions:
1. Place the chicken breasts between 2 sheets of plastic wrap and pound them with a meat mallet until ½ inch thick.

2. Sprinkle salt and pepper over the chicken. Sprinkle flour over the chicken.

3. Place a large skillet over medium flame. To spread the oil, add about a tablespoon of oil and swirl in the pan.

4. In the pan, put as many pieces of chicken as possible. Sear the chicken on both the sides until golden brown. Remove the chicken from the pan placed on a plate using a slotted spoon.

5. In the same way, cook the remaining chicken, adding more oil if needed.

6. Add 2 tablespoons oil into the skillet. When the oil is heated, add mushrooms and cook until brown.

7. Stir in garlic and shallots. Stir-fry for 1 and add salt and pepper to taste. – 2 minutes.

8. Add wine, broth and chicken along with the released juice and cook until the liquid in the pan is half its original quantity.

9. Garnish with parsley and serve along with sautéed spinach or any other sautéed greens of your choice.

Nutrition: Calories: 90 Sodium: 20mg Fat: 3g Cholesterol: 2mg Carbohydrates: 11g Protein: 3g

15. Turkey Apple Burgers

Preparation time: 15 minutes
Cooking time: 8 – 10 minutes
Servings: 2

Ingredients:
1 green apple, cored, peeled, halved
A handful fresh thyme or sage, minced
Pepper to taste
½ teaspoon onion powder
¼ teaspoon garlic powder
Salt to taste
1 teaspoon olive oil
½ pound 93% lean ground turkey
Whole-wheat burger buns or lettuce cups to serve

Directions:
1. Grate one half of the apple and cut the other half into thin slices.

2. Combine grated apple, spices, salt, sage and turkey in a bowl and mix well.

3. Make 2 equal portions of the mixture. Shape into patties.

4. Place a skillet over medium flame. Brush both sides of the patties with oil and put in the tub.

5. Cook until the underside is brown. Turn the burgers over and cook the other side until brown.

6. Serve burgers over buns or lettuce cups. Place sliced apples on top of the burgers and serve.

Nutrition: Calories: 10 218 215 Total Fat: 15 613 Saturated Fat: 3753 Sodium: 1342 Total Carbohydrate: Protein: 121

16. Turkey Sandwiches with Apple and Walnut Mayo

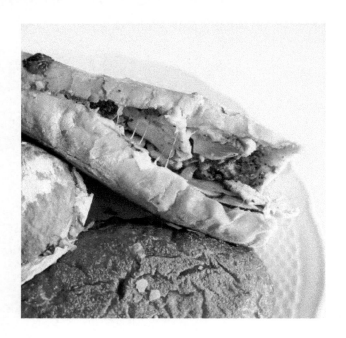

Preparation time: 15 minutes
Cooking time: 4 minutes
Servings: 2

Ingredients:

For walnut mayonnaise:

2 tablespoons finely chopped walnuts

3 – 4 tablespoons mayonnaise

½ tablespoon Dijon mustard

½ tablespoon chopped, fresh parsley

For sandwich:

4 slices whole-wheat bread

½ green apple, peeled, cored, cut into thin slices

Cooked, sliced turkey, as required

A handful rockets

Directions:

1. To make walnut mayonnaise: Combine walnuts, mayonnaise, mustard and parsley in a bowl.

2. Smear walnut mayonnaise on one side of the bread slices.

3. Place arugula on 2 bread slices, on the mayo side. Place turkey slices over it followed by apple slices.

4. Complete the sandwich by covering with remaining bread slices, with mayo side facing down.

5. Cut into desired shape and serve.

Nutrition: Calories: 205 Protein: 5.2g Carbs: 30.7g Fat: 12.1g Sodium: 66. 5mg

17. Sautéed Turkey with Tomatoes and Cilantro

Preparation time: 10 minutes
Cooking time: 15 minutes
Servings: 2 – 3

Ingredients:
½ pound lean ground turkey
½ cup chopped yellow or red onion
Pepper to taste
1 teaspoon olive oil
1 jalapeño or to taste, chopped
½ tablespoon minced garlic
¼ cup chopped tomatoes
¼ teaspoon ground cumin
2 teaspoons red pepper flakes
½ cup chopped fresh cilantro
Salt to taste
A handful parsley leaves

Directions:
1. Place a skillet over medium flame. Add oil and wait before it heats up. Add garlic and sauté for about a minute until light brown.

2. Stir in onions, tomatoes, jalapeño, parsley and red pepper flakes and cook for 4-5 minutes.

3. Stir the turkey and cook until the mixture is brown, breaking the turkey as it cooks.

4. Add cilantro, salt and pepper and stir.

5. Serve hot.

Nutrition: Calories: 416 cal. – kcal: 1750 - Fat: 19 g - Protein: 45 g - Carbs: 28 g - Sodium: 171.5 mg

18. Prawn & Coconut Curry

Preparation Time: 15 Minutes

Cooking Time: 40 Minutes Servings: 1

Ingredients

400g (14oz) tinned chopped tomatoes

400g (14oz) large prawns (shrimps), shelled and raw

25g (1oz) fresh coriander (cilantro) chopped

3 red onions, finely chopped

3 cloves of garlic, crushed

2 bird's eye chillies

½ teaspoon ground coriander (cilantro)

½ teaspoon turmeric

400mls (14fl oz) coconut milk

1 tablespoons olive oil

Juice of 1 lime

Directions

1. Place the onions, garlic, tomatoes, chilis, lime juice, turmeric, ground coriander (cilantro), chillies and half of the fresh coriander (cilantro) into a blender and blitz until you have a smooth curry paste. In a frying pan, heat the olive oil, add the paste and cook for 2 minutes. Stir in the coconut milk and warm it thoroughly. Add the prawns (shrimps) to the paste and cook them until they have turned pink and are completely cooked. Stir in the fresh coriander (cilantro). Serve with rice.

19. Orecchiette with Sausage and Chicory

Preparation time: 10 minutes
Cooking time: 20 – 25 minutes
Servings: 3

Ingredients:
½ pound Orecchiette

½ pound sweet Italian sausage, discard casings

¼ teaspoon crushed red pepper

Salt to taste

2 tablespoons grated pecorino + extra to garnish

2 tablespoons extra-virgin olive oil

1 clove garlic, peeled, thinly sliced

½ pound chicory or escarole, chopped

½ cup chicken stock

A handful fresh mint leaves, chopped

Directions:
1. Cook pasta following the package instructions, adding salt while cooking.

2. Place a large skillet over medium flame. Send the oil a tablespoon and let it heat up.

3. Once oil is heated, add sausage and cook until brown. Break it while it cooks.

4. With a slotted spoon, remove the sausage and put it on a plate.

5. Add a tablespoon of oil. Add garlic and red pepper when the oil is hot, and stir for a few seconds until you get a nice aroma.

6. Stir in chicory and salt and cook covered, until they turn limp. It should take a couple of minutes.

7. Uncover and continue cooking until tender.

8. Add pasta, sausage, cheese and stock and cook until the sauce is slightly thick. Add mint and stir.

9. Serve hot.

Nutrition: 700 Calories 46 g Protein 25 g Carbohydrate 21 g Fat 14 g Saturated Fat 12 mg Cholesterol 93 mg Sodium

20. Lamb and Black Bean Chili

Preparation time: 10 minutes
Cooking time: 1 hour and 30 minutes
Servings: 4

Ingredients:
¾ pound lean ground lamb
1 clove garlic, minced
½ cup dry red wine
1 teaspoon ground cumin
Salt to taste
Hot sauce to taste (optional)
½ cup chopped red onion
1 can (14.1 ounces) whole tomatoes, with its liquid, chopped
½ tablespoon chili powder
1 teaspoon dried oregano
1 ½ cans (15 ounces each) black beans, drained
½ teaspoon sugar
Fresh cilantro sprigs (optional)

Directions:
1. Place a Dutch oven over medium flame. Add lamb, onion and garlic and sauté until brown. Break it while you stir.

2. Use a slotted spoon to remove the mixture and place it on a board lined with paper towels. Discard the remaining fat in the pan. Wipe the pot clean.

3. Place the pot over medium flame. Add tomatoes, spices, oregano and salt and stir. Heat thoroughly.

4. Lower the heat and cook covered, for an hour. Add beans and hot sauce and stir.

5. Cover and simmer for about 30 minutes.

6. Sprinkle cilantro on top and serve.

Nutrition: Calories 270 Fat 13 g Cholesterol 15 mg Sodium 679 mg Potassium 696 mg Carbohydrates 15 g Fiber 6 g Sugar 4 g Protein 19 g

21. Tomato, Bacon and Arugula Quiche with Sweet Potato Crust

Preparation time: 15 minutes - **Cooking time:** 50 minutes- **Servings**: 8

Ingredients:
4 cups shredded sweet potato or yam

Salt to taste

1 red onion, chopped

2 large handfuls baby arugula

12 eggs

2 tablespoons olive oil

8 slices bacon, chopped

16 cherry tomatoes, quartered

6 cloves garlic, minced

Pepper to taste

1 tablespoon butter or ghee

Directions:
1. To make sweet potato crusts: You can grate the sweet potatoes on a box grater or in the food processor.

2. Squeeze excess moisture from the sweet potatoes.

3. Grease 2 pie pans (9 inches each) with some of the olive oil.

4. Add butter, pepper and salt into the bowl of sweet potatoes and mix well. Press the mixture onto the bottom and a little on the sides of the pie pan.
5. Bake the crusts in an oven preheated to 450° F, for around 20 minutes or until golden brown at the edges.

6. Remove the pie crusts from the oven.

7. Meanwhile, place a skillet over medium heat. Add bacon and cook until crisp. Place the bacon on a plate lined with paper towels with a slotted spoon. Discard the fat.

8. Add remaining oil into the skillet. Once oil is heated, add onions and sauté until it turns soft.

9. Stir in tomatoes and arugula and cook until the tomatoes are slightly soft.

10. Add in the garlic and cook for half a minute or so. Turn off the heat. Cool for a while.

11. Meanwhile, crack the eggs into a bowl. Add salt and pepper and whisk well.

12. Add the slightly cooled vegetables and bacon and stir.

13. Divide the egg mixture equally and pour over the baked sweet potato crust.

14. Place the crusts in the oven until the eggs are set, and bake.

15. Let it rest for 10 minutes.

16. Cut each into 4 wedges and serve.

Nutrition: Calories, 515 fat, 30g total carbohydrate, 6g fiber, 657mg sodium, 99g protein.

22. Pomegranate Guacamole

Preparation time: 10 Minutes
Cooking Time: 40 Minutes
Servings 4

Ingredients
Flesh of 2 ripe avocados
Seeds from 1 pomegranate
1 bird's-eye chili pepper, finely chopped ½ red onion, finely chopped
Juice of 1 lime
151 calories per serving

Directions
1. Place the avocado, onion, chill and lime juice into a blender and process until smooth. Stir in the pomegranate seeds. Chill before serving. Serve as a dip for chop vegetables.

23. Broccoli and Beef Stir-Fry

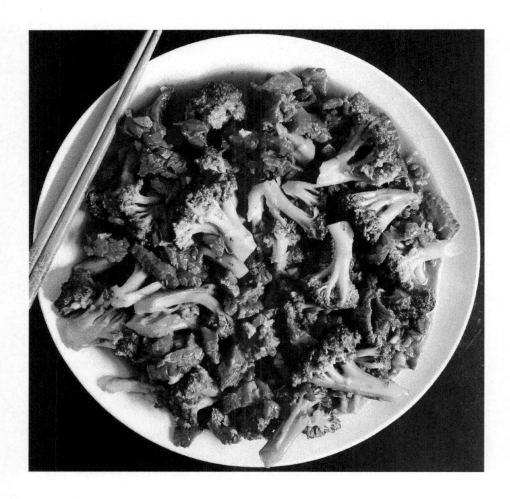

Preparation Time: 5 minutes
Cooking Time: 18 minutes
Servings: 4

Ingredients:

12 ounces frozen broccoli, thawed

Sirloin beef, 8 ounces, sliced into thin strips

1 medium Roma tomato, chopped

1 teaspoon minced garlic

1 tablespoon cornstarch

2 tablespoons soy sauce, reduced-sodium

¼ cup chicken broth, low-sodium

2 tablespoons peanut oil

2 cups cooked brown rice

Directions:

1. Take a frying pan, place it over medium heat, add oil and when hot, add garlic and cook for 1 minute until fragrant.

2. Add vegetable blend, cook for 5 minutes, then transfer vegetable blend to a plate and set aside until needed.

3. Add beef strips into the pan, and then cook for 7 minutes until cooked to the desired level.

4. Prepare the sauce by putting cornstarch in a bowl, and then whisking in soy sauce and broth until well combined.

5. Returned vegetables to the pan, add tomatoes, drizzle with sauce, stir well until coated, And cook until the sauce has thickened, for 2 minutes.

6. Serve with brown rice.

Nutrition: Calories: 373 kcal Total Fat: 17 g Saturated Fat: 0 g Cholesterol: 42 mg Sodium: 351 mg Total Carbs: 37 g Fiber: 5.1 g Sugar: 0 g Protein: 18 g

24. Meatballs with Eggplant

Preparation Time: 15 minutes
Cooking Time: 60 minutes
Servings: 6

Ingredients:
1-pound ground beef
½ cup green bell pepper, chopped
2 medium eggplants, peeled and diced
½ teaspoon minced garlic
1 cup stewed tomatoes
½ cup white onion, diced
1/3 cup canola oil
1 teaspoon lemon and pepper seasoning, salt-free
1 teaspoon turmeric
1 teaspoon Mrs. Dash seasoning blend
2 cups of water

Directions:
1. Take a large skillet pan, place it over medium heat, add oil in it and when hot, add garlic and green bell pepper and cook for 4 minutes until sauté.

2. Transfer the mixture of green pepper to a plate, set aside until required, then place the pieces of eggplant in the pan and cook until browned for 4 minutes per side and, when finished, transfer the eggplant to a plate and set aside until necessary.

3. Take a medium bowl, place beef in it, add onion, season with all the spices, Shape the mixture into 30 small meatballs and stir until well combined.

4. Place meatballs into the pan in a single layer and cook for 3 minutes, or until browned.

5. When done, place all the meatballs in the pan, add cooked bell pepper mixture in it along with eggplant, stir in water and tomatoes and simmer for 30 minutes at low heat setting until thoroughly cooked.

6. Serve straight away.

Nutrition: Calories: 265 kcal Total Fat: 18 g Saturated Fat: 0 g Cholesterol: 47 mg Sodium: 153 mg Total Carbs: 12 g Fiber: 4.6 g Protein: 17 g

25. Slow-Cooked Lemon Chicken

Preparation Time: 20 minutes
Cooking Time: 7 hours
Servings: 4

Ingredients:
1 teaspoon dried oregano
¼ teaspoon ground black pepper
2 tablespoons butter, unsalted
1-pound chicken breast, boneless, skinless
¼ cup chicken broth, low sodium
¼ cup water
1 tablespoon lemon juice
2 cloves garlic, minced
1 teaspoon fresh basil, chopped

Directions:
1. In a small bowl, combine the oregano and ground black pepper. Rub the chicken with the mixture.

2. In a medium-size skillet over medium heat, melt the butter. In the melted butter, brown the chicken and then move the chicken to the slow cooker.

3. In the skillet, placed the chicken broth, water, lemon juice and garlic. Bring it to a boil so the browned bits are loosened from the skillet. Pour the chicken over it.

4. Cover, set the slow cooker for 2½ hours on high or 5 hours on low.

5. Add basil and baste chicken. Cover, cook on high for an additional 15–30 minutes or until chicken is tender.

Nutrition: Calories: 197 kcal Total Fat: 9 g Saturated Fat: 5 g Cholesterol: 99mg Sodium: 57 mg Total Carbs: 1 g Fiber: 0.3 g Sugar: 0 g Protein: 26 g

26. Pork with Pak Choi

Preparation Time: 15 Minutes

Cooking Time: 10 Minutes

Servings: 4

Ingredients

100g of shiitake mushrooms, sliced

1 tablespoon of corn flour

200g pak choi or choi sum-cut into thin slices 125ml of chicken stock

1 tablespoon of tomato purée

1 teaspoon of brown sugar

1 clove garlic, peeled and crushed

1 shallot, peeled and sliced

100g of bean sprouts

1 tablespoon of water

400g of pork mince (10% fat)

1 thumb (5cm) fresh ginger -peeled and grated 400g of firm tofu, cut into large cubes

1 tablespoon of rice wine

1 tablespoon of soy sauce

A large handful (20g) of parsley, chopped 1 tablespoon of rapeseed oil

Directions

1. Place the tofu on kitchen paper, cover it with kitchen paper, and then set it aside.

2. Mix the water and corn flour in a small bowl and remove the lumps.Add in rice wine, brown sugar, chicken stock,tomato puree, and soy sauce. Also, add in the crushed ginger and garlic them mix.

3. Place a large frying pan or wok on high heat and add oil to it. Add the mushrooms and stir-fry for 2 to 3 minutes until cooked and glossy. Using a slotted spoon, remove the mushrooms from the pan and let them rest. Add tofu to the pan, fry it until it is brown on all sides, when finished and set aside, extract it with a slotted spoon.

4. Add the pak choi to your pan or wok, and stir-fry for about 2 minutes and, then add the mince. Cook it until it's cooked and then add the sauce to it. Reduce the heat by a notch and allow 12 minutes for the sauce to bubble around the meat.

5. Add the tofu, beansprouts, and mushrooms to the pan and warm them all through. Remove it from the heat andmix in parsley then serve right away.

27. Chicken stir-fry

Ingredients

150g (5oz) egg noodles

50g (2oz) cauliflower flore ts, roughly chopped 25g (1oz) kale, finely chopped 25g (1oz) mange tout

2 sticks of celery, finely chopped 2 chicken breasts

1 red pepper (bell pepper), chopped 1 clove of garlic

2 tablespoons soy sauce

100mls (3½ fl oz) chicken stock (broth) 1 tablespoon olive oil

Servings 2

566 calories per serving

Directions

1.   As per the instructions, cook the noodles and set them aside to keep warm. Heat the oil in a wok or a frying pan and add the garlic and chicken. Add in the kale, celery, cauliflower, red pepper (bell pepper), mange tout and cook for 4 minutes. Pour in the chicken stock (broth) and soy sauce and cook for 3 minutes or until the chicken is thoroughly cooked. Stir in the cooked noodles and serve.

28. Tuna with lemon herb dressing

Preparation time: 5 Minutes

Cooking Time: 15 Minutes

Servings: 4

Ingredients

4 tuna steaks 1 tablespoon olive oil For the dressing:

25g (1oz) pitted green olives, chopped 2 tablespoons fresh parsley, chopped 1 tablespoon fresh basil, chopped 2 tablespoons olive oil Freshly squeezed juice of 1 lemon Servings 4 241 calories per serving

Directions

1.   In a griddle pan, heat a tablespoon of olive oil. Add the tuna steaks and cook on a high heat for 2-3 minutes on each side. Reduce the cooking time if you want them rare. Place the dressing ingredients into a bowl and mix them well. Serve the tuna steaks with a dollop of dressing over them. Serve alongside a leafy rocket salad.

29. Kale, apple & fennel soup

Preparation time: 5 Minutes

Cooking Time: 20 Minutes

Servings: 4

Ingredients

450g (1lb) kale, chopped

200g (7oz) fennel, chopped

2 apples, peeled, cored and chopped 2 tablespoons fresh parsley, chopped 1 tablespoon olive oil

Sea salt

Freshly ground black pepper

Directions

1. In a saucepan, heat the oil, add the kale and fennel and cook for 5 minutes until the fennel softens. Stir in the parsley and apples. Cover and bring to a boil with hot water, and simmer for 10 minutes. Use a hand blender or blitz for food processing until the soup is smooth. With salt and pepper, season.

30. Lentil soup

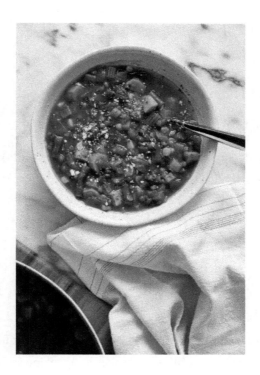

Preparation time: 5 Minutes

Cooking Time: 25 Minutes

Servings: 4

Ingredients

175g (6oz) red lentils

1 red onion, chopped

1 clove of garlic, chopped

2 sticks of celery, chopped

2 carrots, chopped

½ bird's-eye chilli

1 teaspoon ground cumin

1 teaspoon ground turmeric

1 teaspoon ground coriander (cilantro) 1200mls (2 pints) vegetable stock (broth) 2 tablespoons olive oil

Sea salt

Freshly ground black pepper

Directions

1. In a saucepan, heat the oil and add the onion and cook for 5 minutes. Put the carrots, lentils, celery, chilli, cilantro, cumin, turmeric, and garlic in the mixture and cook for 5 minutes. Pour the stock (broth) in, bring it to a boil, reduce the heat and simmer for 45 minutes. Purée the soup until smooth, using a hand blender or food processor. With salt and pepper, season. Just serve.

31. Cauliflower & walnut soup

Preparation time: 5 Minutes

Cooking Time: 15 Minutes

Servings: 4

Ingredients

450g (1lb) cauliflower, chopped 8 w alnut halves, chopped

1 red onion, chopped

900mls (1½ pints) vegetable stock (broth) 100mls (3½ fl oz)

double cream (heavy cream) ½ teaspoon turmeric

1 tablespoon olive oil

Directions

1.   Heat the oil in a saucepan, add the cauliflower and red onion, and then cook, stirring continuously, for 4 minutes. Pour (broth) into the stock, bring to a boil and cook for 15 minutes. Stir in the turmeric, double cream and walnuts. Process the soup until smooth and fluffy, using a food processor or hand blender. Serve in bowls with a sprinkling of sliced walnuts and top off.

32. Celery & blue cheese soup

Preparation time: 5 Minutes

Cooking Time: 25 Minutes

Servings: 4

Ingredients

125g (4oz) blue cheese

25g (1oz) butter

1 head of celery (approx 65 0g) 1 red onion, chopped

900mls (1½ pints) chicken stock (broth) 150mls (5fl oz) single cream

Directions

1.   In a saucepan, heat the butter, add the onion and celery, and then cook until the vegetables soften. Pour the stock in, bring it to a boil, then reduce the heat and simmer for 15 minutes. Pour in the milk until it has melted and stir in the cheese. Serve right away and eat.

33. Spicy squash soup

Preparation time: 5 Minutes

Cooking Time: 35 Minutes

Servings: 4

Ingredients

150g (5oz) kale

1 butternut squash, peeled, de-seeded and chopped 1 red onion, chopped

3 bird's-eye chillies, chopped 3 cloves of garlic

2 teaspoons turmeric

1 teaspoon ground ginger

600mls (1 pint) vegetable stock (broth) 2 tablespoons olive oil

calories per serving

Directions

1.   In a saucepan, heat the olive oil, add the chopped butternut squash and onion and cook until tender, for 6 minutes. Add kale, garlic, chilli, turmeric and ginger and cook, stirring constantly, for 2 minutes. Bring it to a boil in the vegetable stock (broth) and simmer for 20 minutes. Use a food processor or a hand blender to smoothly process it. Serve alone or with a cream or crème fraiche swirl. Enjoy.

34. French onion soup

Preparation time: 5 Minutes

Cooking Time: 25 Minutes

Servings: 4

Ingredients

750g (1¾ lbs) red onions, thinly sliced 50g (2oz) cheddar cheese, grated (shredded) 12g (½ oz) butter

2 teaspoons flour

2 slices wholemeal bread

900mls (1½ pints) beef stock (broth) 1 tablespoon olive oil

Directions

1. Heat the butter and oil in a large pan. Attach the onions and cook gently for 25 minutes on a low heat, stirring occasionally. Attach the flour and whisk well. Pour in and keep stirring in the stock (broth). Boil, minimize heat and simmer for 30 minutes. Bring to a boil. Cut the slices of bread into triangles, sprinkle with cheese and place them under a hot grill (broiler) until the cheese has melted. Serve the soup into bowls and add 2 triangles of cheesy toast on top. Enjoy.

35. Cream of broccoli & kale soup

Preparation time: 5 Minutes

Cooking Time: 35 Minutes

Servings: 4

Ingredients

250g (9oz) broccoli

250g (9oz) kale

1 potato, peeled and chopped

1 red onion, chopped

600mls (1 pint) vegetable stock 300mls (½ pint) milk

1 tablespoon olive oil

Sea salt

 Freshly ground black pepper

Directions

1.   In a saucepan, heat the olive oil, add the onion and cook for 5 minutes. Put the potato, kale and broccoli into the mixture and cook for 5 minutes. Pour the stock (broth) and milk in and boil for 20 minutes. Process the soup until smooth and fluffy, using a food processor or hand blender. With salt and pepper, season. Re-heat and serve if desired.

36. Sesame miso chicken

Preparation time: 5 Minutes

Cooking Time: 40 Minutes

Servings 3

Ingredients:

1 skinless cod fillet

½ cup buckwheat

½ red onion, sliced

2 stalks celery, sliced

10 green beans

2 cups kale, roughly chopped

3 sprigs of parsley

1 garlic clove, finely chopped

1 pinch cayenne or ½ chilli

1 tsp. Finely chopped fresh ginger

1 tsp. Sesame seeds

2 teaspoons of miso

1 tbsp. Mirin/ rice wine vinegar

1 tbsp. Extra virgin olive oil

1 tbsp. Of soy sauce 1 tsp ground turmeric

Directions:

1. Coat the cod with a mixture of the miso, mirin and 1 teaspoon of the oil and set aside for 30 minutes up to one hour in the refrigerator.

2. Heat the oven to 400 f, then bake the cod for 10 minutes.

3. Sautee the onion and stir-fry in the oil that remains along with the green beans, kale, celery, chili pepper, garlic, ginger. Sautee until the kale is wilted but the beans and celery are tender. Add dashes of water if needed to the pan as you go.

4. Cook the buckwheat for 3 minutes with the turmeric according to the product instructions. To stir-fry, add the sesame seeds, parsley and tamari and serve with the greens and fish.

37. Sirt Salmon Salad

Preparation time: 5 Minutes - Cooking Time: 30 Minutes - Servings 1

Ingredients

1 large Medjool date, pitted then chopped

50g of chicory leaves

50g of rocket

1 tablespoon of extra-virgin olive oil

10g of parsley, chopped

10g of celery leaves, chopped

40g of celery, sliced

15g of walnuts, chopped

1 tablespoon of capers

20g of red onions-sliced

80g of avocado-peeled, stoned, and sliced Juice of ¼ lemon

100g of smoked salmon slices alternatives: lentils, tinned tuna, or cooked chicken breast

Directions

1.   On a large plate, place all the salad leaves, then mix the rest of the ingredients and spread evenly on top of the leaves.

38. Red Onion Dhal

Preparation Time: 45 Minutes

Serves 4

Ingredients

1 tsp extra virgin olive oil

1 tsp mustard seeds

40g red onion, finely chopped

1 garlic clove, finely chopped

1 tsp finely chopped fresh ginger

1 bird's eye chili, finely chopped

1 tsp mild curry powder

2 tsp ground turmeric

300ml vegetable stock

40g red lentils, rinsed

50g kale

50ml tinned coconut milk

50g buckwheat

Directions

1.   In a moderately sized sauce pan, warm the olive oil over a medium heat. Using the mustard seeds to ossify and fry until they begin to crackle. Add the

garlic, ginger, chili and onion frying for 10 minutes, or until the onion is tender.

2.   Throw in 1 tsp turmeric and curry powder, and then stir. Cook until fragrant for a few minutes, then pour in the

3.   stock and bring to the boil. Pour in the lentils and cook for 30 minutes.

4.   Add the coconut milk and kale, cooking for another 5 minutes or so. As the dhal is brewing, rinse the buckwheat with water and cook it according to packet Directions . Drain and serve with the dhal.

39. Tofu & Shiitake mushroom soup

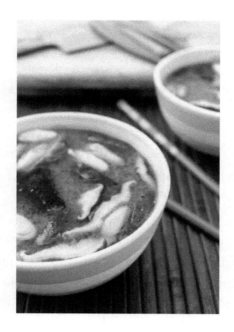

Preparation Time: 15 Minutes

Serves 4

Ingredients

10g dried wakame

1L vegetable stock

200g shiitake mushrooms, sliced

120g miso paste

1* 400g firm tofu, diced

2 green onion, trimmed and diagonally chopped

1 bird's eye chili, finely chopped

Directions

1.   Soak the wakame in lukewarm water for 10-15 minutes before draining.

2.   In a medium-sized saucepan add the vegetable stock and bring to the boil. Toss in the mushrooms and simmer for 23 minutes.

3.   Mix miso paste with 3-4 tbsp of vegetable stock from the saucepan, until the miso is entirely dissolved. Pour the miso-stock back into the pan and add the tofu, wakame, green onions and chili, then serve immediately.

40. Chicken Soup

Preparation Time: 25 Minutes

Cooking Time: 60 Minutes

 Servings: 4

Ingredients

1 teaspoon of smoked paprika

300ml passata

Salt and freshly ground black pepper

1 teaspoon of dried mixed herbs

1 x 400g can of black beans, drained

2 cloves garlic, peeled and crushed

1 carrot, peeled and roughly chopped

1 liter of water

1 teaspoon of mild chili powder

1 red chili, deseeded then finely chopped ½ teaspoon of turmeric

30g (large handful) of flat leaf parsley, chopped 1 x 400g can chopped tomatoes

1 teaspoon of paprika

½ teaspoon of ground cumin

1 green pepper, deseeded and chopped

1 x 400g can kidney beans, drained

4 chicken drumsticks

2 shallots, peeled then roughly chopped

Directions

1.   Take a large saucepan and add in the chicken drumsticks, carrot, and shallots. Pour in the water and let it simmer.

2.   Enable 20 minutes to cook, then with a spoon (slotted) remove the chicken drumsticks and set aside to cool.

3.   Add in the chopped tomatoes, garlic, passata, chili, and green pepper, and let it simmer again. Put in the driedherbs, paprika, turmeric, smoked paprika, chili powder, and cumin, then simmer again for 30 minutes.

4.   Pull off the skin from the chicken then pinch as much chicken as possible from the bone. Shred the chicken meat,place it on the pan along with the kidney beans and black beans, and cook for five minutes.

5.   Remove from the sun, add and mix in the parsley. Season with salt and pepper (to taste).

41. Chicken curry with potatoes and kale

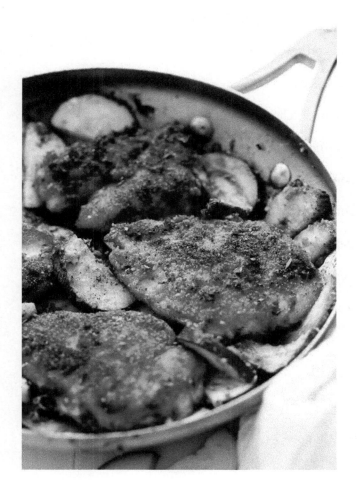

Preparation time: 10 Minutes

Cooking Time: 20 Minutes

Servings: 4

Ingredients

600g chicken breast, cut into pieces

4 tablespoons of extra virgin olive oil

3 tablespoons turmeric

2 red onions, sliced

2 red chilies, finely chopped

3 cloves of garlic, finely chopped

1 tablespoon freshly chopped ginger

1 tablespoon curry powder

1 tin of small tomatoes (400ml)

500ml chicken broth

200ml coconut milk

2 pieces cardamom

1 cinnamon stick

600g potatoes mainly waxy)

10g parsley, chopped

175g kale, chopped

5g coriander, chopped

Directions

1. Marinate the chicken in a teaspoon of olive oil and a tablespoon of turmeric for about 30 minutes. Then fry in a high frying pan at high heat for about 4 minutes. Remove from the pan and set aside.

2. In a pan with chili, garlic, onion and onion, heat a tablespoon of oil.

From ginger. Boil all over medium heat, add the curry powder and a tablespoon of turmeric and cook, stirring occasionally, for another two minutes. Add tomatoes, cook for another two minutes until finally chicken stock, coconut milk, cardamom and cinnamon stick are added. Cook for about 45 to 60 minutes and add some broth if necessary.

3. In the meantime, preheat the oven to 425 °. Peel and chop the potatoes. Bring water to the boil, add the potatoes with turmeric and cook for 5 minutes. Then pour off the water and let it evaporate for about 10 minutes. Spread olive oil together with the potatoes on a baking tray and bake in the oven for 30 minutes.

4. When the potatoes and curry are almost ready, add the coriander, kale and chicken and cook for five minutes until the chicken is hot.

5. Add parsley to the potatoes and serve with the chicken curry.

42. Paleo Chocolate Wraps with Fruits

Preparation time: 25 minutes

Cooking time: 0 minutes

Servings: 2

Ingredients:

4 pieces Egg

100 ml Almond milk

2 tablespoons Arrowroot powder

4 tablespoons Chestnut flour

1 tablespoon Olive oil (mild)

2 tablespoons Maple syrup

2 tablespoons Cocoa powder

1 tablespoon Coconut oil

1-piece Banana

2 pieces Kiwi (green)

2 pieces Mandarins

Directions:

1. Mix all ingredients (except fruit and coconut oil) into an even dough.

2. Melt some coconut oil in a small pan and pour a quarter of the batter into it.

3. Bake it like a pancake baked on both sides.

4. Place the fruit in a wrap and serve it lukewarm.

5. A wonderfully sweet start to the day!

43. Sirt Energy Balls

Preparation Time: 10 Minutes

Cooking Time: 40 Minutes

Servings: 20 balls

Ingredients

1 mug of mixed nuts (with plenty of walnuts) 7 Medjool dates

1 tablespoon of coconut oil

2 tablespoons of cocoa powder Zest of 1 orange (optional)

Directions

1.   Start by placing the nuts in a food processor and grind them until almost powdered (more or less depending on thepreferred texture of your energy balls).

2.   Add the Medjool dates, coconut oil, cacao powder, and run the blender again until fully mixed. Place the blend ina refrigerator for half an hour, and then shape them into balls. You can add in the zest of an orange as you blend.

44. Kale and Tofu Curry

Preparation Time: 15 Minutes

Cooking Time: 40 Minutes

Servings: 12

Ingredients

1 red chili, deseeded and thinly sliced

1 teaspoon of salt

1 liter of boiling water

1 large onion, chopped

½ teaspoon of ground turmeric

200g of firm tofu, chopped into cubes

¼ teaspoon of cayenne pepper

4 cloves of garlic, peeled then grated

200g of kale leaves, stalks removed and torn ½ teaspoon of ground cumin

250g of dried red lentils

1 large thumb fresh ginger (about 7cm peeled then grated)

1 teaspoon of paprika

2 tomatoes, roughly chopped

Juice of 1 lime

1 tablespoon of rapeseed oil

50g frozen soya edamame beans

Directions

1.   Place a pan over low heat and add oil to it. Add in the onions and cook for five minutes, then add in chili, garlic,and ginger and cook for two more minutes. Add the salt, cayenne, paprika, turmeric, and cumin. Stir through then add in the red lentils and stir again.

2.   Pour in boiling water and simmer for 10 minutes.

3.   Reduce the heat and let it cook for another 20 to 30 minutes until the curry has the consistency of thick porridge.Add the soya beans, tomatoes, and tofu and let it cook for 5 minutes. Add the kale leaves, lime juice, and let it cook until the kale is tender. Serve.

45. Bean Stew

Preparation Time: 25 Minutes

Cooking Time: 40 Minutes

Servings: 4

Ingredients

50g of kale, chopped roughly

½ bird's eye chili, chopped finely (optional) 40g of buckwheat 50g of red onion, chopped finely

1 garlic clove, chopped finely

1 tablespoon of roughly chopped parsley 200ml vegetable stock

1 teaspoon of Herbes de Provence

200g of tinned mixed beans

1 teaspoon of tomato purée

1 x 400g tin of chopped Italian tomatoes

30g celery, trimmed and chopped finely

1 tablespoon of extra-virgin olive oil

30g of carrot, peeled and chopped finely

Directions

1. Heat oil over medium-low heat in a medium-sized saucepan. Add in the onion, celery, chili, carrot,garlic and herbs (if using) until the onions are soft enough but not colored.

2. Add the stock, tomato purée, and tomatoes and bring to a boil.

3. Put in the beans and allow for 30 minutes simmering.

4. Add the kales and cook for 5-10 minutes or until the kale is tender, and then add in parsley.

5. As it cools, cook the buckwheat as per the Directions on the packet. Drain the buckwheat and serve with thecooked stew.

46. Sirt Salmon Salad

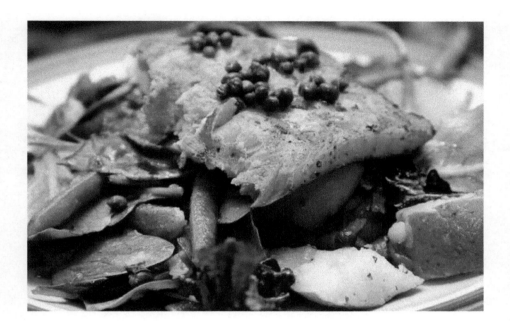

Preparation Time: 10 Minutes

Cooking Time: 10 Minutes

Servings: 1

Ingredients

1 large Medjool date, pitt ed then chopped

50g of chicory leaves

50g of rocket

1 tablespoon of extra-virgin olive oil

10g of parsley, chopped

10g of celery leaves, chopped

40g of celery, sliced

15g of walnuts, chopped

1 tablespoon of capers

20g of red onions-sliced

80g of avocado-peeled, stoned, and sliced Juice of ¼ lemon

100g of smoked salmon slices (alternatives: lentils, tinned tuna, or cooked chicken breast)

Directions

1.   On a large plate, place all the salad leaves, then combine the remaining ingredients and spread evenly on top of the leaves.

47. Roasted vegetable salad

Preparation time: 5 Minutes

Cooking Time: 20 Minutes

Servings: 4-5

Ingredients:

3 tomatoes, halved

1 zucchini, quartered

1 fennel bulb, thinly sliced

2 small eggplants, ends trimmed, quartered

1 large red pepper, halved, deseeded, cut into strips

2 medium onions, quartered

1 tsp oregano

2 tbsp extra virgin olive oil

For the dressing

2/3 cup yogurt

1 tbsp fresh lemon juice1 small garlic clove, chopped

Directions:

1.   Place the zucchini, eggplant, pepper, fennel, onions, tomatoes and olive oil on a lined baking sheet. Season with salt, pepper and oregano and cook in an oven at 500 degrees F until golden, about 20 minutes.

2.   Whisk the yogurt, lemon juice and garlic in a bowl. Taste and season with salt and pepper. Divide the vegetables in 4-5 plates. Top with the yogurt mixture and serve.

48. Warm leek and sweet potato salad

Preparation time: 5 Minutes

Cooking Time: 30 Minutes

Servings: 4-5

Ingredients:

1.5lb sweet potato, unpeeled, cut into 1-inch pieces

4 small leeks, trimmed and cut into 1-inch slices

5-6 white mushrooms, halved

1 cup baby arugula le aves

2 tbsp extra virgin olive oil

For the dressing

½ cup yogurt 1 tbsp dijon mustard

Directions:

1.   Preheat oven to 350 f. Line a baking tray with baking paper. Place the sweet potato, leeks and mushrooms on the baking tray. Drizzle and toss with olive oil to coat. Roast until golden or for 20 minutes.

2. In a small bowl or cup, combine your yogurt and mustard. Place vegetables, mushrooms and baby arugula in a salad bowl and toss to combine. Serve drizzled with the yogurt mixture.

49. Chickpeas, Onion, Tomato & Parsley Salad in a Jar

Preparation time: 5 Minutes

Cooking Time: 50 Minutes

Servings 2

Ingredients

1 cup cooked chickpeas

1/2 cup chopped tomatoes

1/2 of a small onion, chopped

1 tbsp. chia seeds

1 Tbsp. chopped parsley

Dressing:

1 tbsp. olive oil and 1 tbsp. of Chlorella. 1 tbsp. fresh lemon juice and pinch of sea salt

Directions:

1.   Put ingredients in this order: dressing, tomatoes, chickpeas, onions and parsley.

50. Kale & Feta Salad with Cranberry Dressing

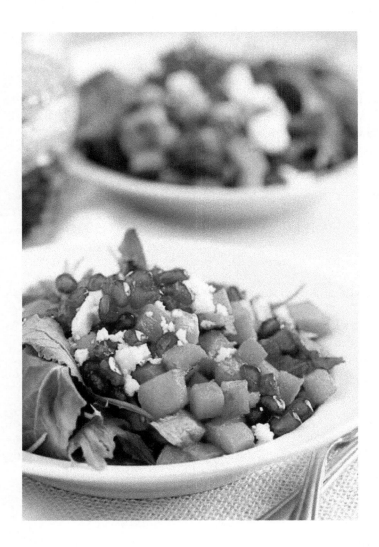

Preparation time: 5 Minutes

Cooking Time: 30 Minutes

Servings 2

Ingredients

9oz kale, finely chopped

2oz walnuts, chopped

3oz feta cheese, crumbled

1 apple, peeled, cored and sliced

4 medjool dates, chopped

For the Dressing

3oz cranberries

½ red onion, chopped

3 tablespoons olive oil

3 tablespoons water

2 teaspoons honey

1 tablespoon red wine vinegar

Sea salt

Directions

1.   In a food processor, place the ingredients for the dressing and process until smooth. You can add a little extra water if appropriate, if it seems too thick. Place all the ingredients in the salad in a bowl. Pour the dressing on and toss the salad into the mixture until it is well covered.

Lightning Source UK Ltd.
Milton Keynes UK
UKHW021441160321
380432UK00001B/26